EVERYTHING ABOUT APLASTIC ANEMIA

A Complete Guide For Patients, Caregivers, And Healthcare Professionals - Causes, Symptoms, Diagnosis, Treatment, Expert Advice, Coping Strategies, And More

DR. CADE JOSUE

Table of Contents

CHAPTER ONE...11

A Brief Overview Of Aplastic Anemia.............11

Comprehending Blood Cells And Bone Marrow
....13

The Following Are The Causes Of Aplastic
Anemia:...14

The Following Are Risk Factors For Aplastic
Anemia:...17

CHAPTER TWO..21

Symptoms And Signs Of Aplastic Anemia.......21

Analytical Procedures For Aplastic Anemia 22

The Categorization Of Aplastic Anemia..........25

The Progression Of Aplastic Anemia 27

CHAPTER THREE 29

Alternatives To Aplastic Anemia Treatment...29

Medications Employed In The Treatment Of
Aplastic Anemia..31

CHAPTER FOUR...35

Management And Supportive Care For Aplastic
Anemia..35

Adverse Reactions And Complications Of Aplastic Anemia.................38

CHAPTER FIVE..................43

Outlook And Prognosis For Patients With Aplastic Anemia..................43

Coping Mechanisms And Lifestyle Choices For Aplastic Anemia..................46

Summary....................50

THE END 52

DISCLAIMER

The information provided in this book is for general informational purposes only. It is not intended as medical advice, diagnosis, or treatment.

The content of this book should not be considered a substitute for professional medical advice. Readers should consult with a qualified healthcare provider for diagnosis and treatment of any medical conditions they have.

While every effort has been made to ensure the accuracy and completeness of the information presented, the author makes no representations or warranties of any kind, express or implied, about the completeness, accuracy, reliability, suitability, or availability with respect to the information, contained in this book.

The author disclaims any responsibility for any loss or damage resulting from reliance on the information provided in this book. References to individuals, products, websites, organizations, or other names are for informational purposes only and do not imply endorsement.

By reading this book, readers acknowledge that they are responsible for their own health decisions and should seek appropriate medical advice when necessary.

ABOUT THIS BOOK

"Everything About Aplastic Anemia" is an essential book for healthcare practitioners, researchers, and individuals in quest of a comprehensive understanding of the complex facets associated with aplastic anemia. This book is organized with great care and precision, functioning as an all-encompassing manual that provides a deep comprehension of this intricate hematological disorder.

The introductory section establishes the foundation by presenting a comprehensive outline of aplastic anemia, clarifying its cause, and delineating the importance of bone marrow and blood cells in the pathophysiological process. Further elaboration is provided in subsequent chapters as the condition's multifaceted causes, risk factors, and an extensive array of symptoms are dissected.

This book provides an overview of the diagnostic landscape, detailing the various tests that are utilized to detect and classify aplastic anemia. Additionally, it streamlines the process of understanding the disease by classifying it into distinct phases and classifications, which is crucial for developing individualized therapeutic approaches.

The discussion revolves around the various treatment modalities that are accessible for aplastic anemia. Every treatment alternative, ranging from traditional pharmaceuticals to innovative techniques such as bone marrow stem cell transplants, is thoroughly examined, providing clinicians with an all-encompassing set of resources to proficiently navigate treatment choices.

Moreover, this book elucidates the critical significance of supportive care in the management of aplastic anemia, including the prevention of complications and the alleviation of adverse effects. It furnishes healthcare providers with indispensable insights regarding prognosis and outlook, enabling them to furnish patients and their families with well-informed guidance and support.

The final sections provide a comprehensive perspective, placing particular emphasis on lifestyle modifications and coping mechanisms as means to improve the overall well-being of people dealing with aplastic anemia. Fundamentally, "Everything About Aplastic Anemia" surpasses its status as a simple reference text and becomes an essential companion on the path to comprehending, controlling, and ultimately overcoming aplastic anemia.

CHAPTER ONE

A Brief Overview Of Aplastic Anemia

Aplastic anemia is an uncommon and critical medical condition distinguished by an insufficiency of all blood cell types, which is the result of inadequate production of blood cells by the bone marrow.

A bone marrow failure disorder in which the marrow does not generate sufficient quantities of platelets, red blood cells, and white blood cells. Vaccine-immune symptoms may vary in intensity from mild to potentially fatal, contingent upon the severity of the ailment.

Bone marrow, the porous tissue contained within bones, is essential for the synthesis of red blood cells. Erythrocytes transport oxygen to the tissues of the body, leukocytes aid in the struggle against infections, and platelets (thrombocytes) facilitate blood coagulation.

Aplastic anemia is characterized by injury to or suppression of the bone marrow, which hinders its capacity to generate these vital blood cells.

Aplastic anemia may manifest in a gradual manner (chronic) or manifest abruptly (acute). Acute instances are generally more severe and may necessitate urgent medical intervention, whereas chronic instances may develop gradually.

While the condition has the potential to impact people of all ages, it is diagnosed with greater frequency among adolescents and young adults. Although aplastic anemia is uncommon, its precise prevalence is challenging to ascertain owing to discrepancies in patient reporting and diagnostic practices.

Comprehending Blood Cells And Bone Marrow

A comprehensive understanding of aplastic anemia necessitates knowledge of the functions of blood cells and the significance of bone marrow.

As an essential constituent of the hematopoietic system, bone marrow is accountable for the lifelong production of blood cells. Long bones, including the femur and humerus, as well as the sternum, ribcage, and pelvis, contain this substance within their internal spaces.

The formation of blood cells, or hematopoiesis, takes place in the bone marrow. Hematopoietic stem cells, which are stem cells, serve as the progenitors of every blood cell. The stem cells exhibit a noteworthy capacity for differentiation into a diverse array of specialized cell subtypes, such as platelets, red blood cells, and white blood cells.

Red blood cells (erythrocytes) are responsible for removing carbon dioxide and transporting oxygen from the lungs to the body's tissues. Leukocytes, which are white blood cells, play a vital role in the immune system by protecting against foreign invaders and infections. Blood coagulation is dependent on platelets (thrombocytes), which prevent excessive hemorrhage in the event of blood vessel injury.

Aplastic anemia is characterized by insufficient production of these blood cells by the bone marrow. Manifestations of this insufficiency may include fatigue, frailty, dyspnea, heightened vulnerability to infections, and proneness to injury or hemorrhaging.

The Following Are The Causes Of Aplastic Anemia:

There are numerous potential causes of aplastic anemia, including environmental stimuli, acquired and inherited factors, and exposure to specific substances. Comprehending these aetiologies is critical for precise diagnosis and effective treatment of the ailment.

1. Autoimmune Disorders: Aplastic anemia may result when the immune system of the body erroneously targets and destroys cells of the bone marrow. Influenza viruses and specific medications are potential triggers for this autoimmune response.

2. Toxin Exposure: Specific toxins, chemicals, or radiation can induce injury to the bone marrow, resulting in its dysfunction and subsequent development of aplastic anemia. Substances that have been identified as potential causes of harm to bone marrow consist of benzene, pesticides, chemotherapy medications, and ionizing radiation.

3. Specific viral infections, including hepatitis, cytomegalovirus (CMV), Epstein-Barr virus

(EBV), and HIV, have been linked to the progression of aplastic anemia. These infections have the potential to induce an autoimmune response that results in bone marrow failure or direct damage to the bone marrow.

4. Genetic Predisposition: Although acquired aplastic anemia is characterized by the onset of the disease in response to environmental factors, a minority of cases might exhibit a genetic element. Although uncommon, individuals may be predisposed to develop aplastic anemia due to inherited genetic mutations.

5. Specific medications, including antibiotics and chemotherapy medicines, have been associated with an increased risk of developing aplastic anemia. These medications can inhibit the function of the bone marrow, resulting in a reduction in blood cell production.

6. Unidentified Causes: Despite exhaustive evaluation, the precise etiology of aplastic anemia may occasionally elude determination. Idiopathic aplastic anemia comprises a substantial proportion of the observed cases.

Aplastic anemia is a multifactorial disorder characterized by a combination of environmental influences, genetic predisposition, and immune dysregulation, among other potential causes. Ascertaining the fundamental etiology of aplastic anemia is critical to optimize patient outcomes and determine the most effective therapeutic strategy.

The Following Are Risk Factors For Aplastic Anemia:

1. Idiopathic Causes: Aplastic anemia is frequently referred to as idiopathic aplastic anemia when the precise etiology is uncertain. This particular form constitutes a substantial proportion of the total number of cases.

2. Acquired Components:

• Chemical Exposure: The risk of developing aplastic anemia can be increased through exposure to specific chemicals, including benzene, pesticides, and certain petrochemicals.

Certain medications, specifically antibiotics and chemotherapy medicines, have the potential to induce aplastic anemia as an adverse effect.

• The administration of high doses of radiation therapy, as in the treatment of cancer, has the potential to induce aplastic anemia by causing injury to the bone marrow.

3. Hereditary Disorders: Fanconi anemia and other inherited forms of aplastic anemia are brought about by genetic mutations that impair the functionality of stem cells in the bone marrow.

4. Specific viral infections, such as hepatitis, Epstein-Barr virus (EBV), and HIV, have been

associated with an elevated susceptibility to aplastic anemia.

5. Autoimmune Disorders: Systemic lupus erythematosus (SLE) and other conditions in which the immune system attacks the body's cells are examples of conditions that can cause aplastic anemia.

CHAPTER TWO

Symptoms And Signs Of Aplastic Anemia

Contingent on the individual's overall health and the severity of the condition, the signs and symptoms of aplastic anemia can vary considerably. Typical indications and symptoms consist of:

1. Anemia, which is characterized by a deficiency of red blood cells, may lead to chronic fatigue and frailty.

2. Oxygen deprivation resulting from a deficiency in red blood cells can cause dyspnea, particularly when engaging in vigorous physical activity.

3. Anemia frequently results in a complexion that is pallid or yellow in color.

4. A diminished white blood cell count elevates the susceptibility to infections, thereby resulting in recurrent ailments and extended periods of recuperation.

5. Prolonged hemorrhage from minor wounds or injuries, simple discoloration, and nosebleeds are all potential complications of low platelet counts.

6. Petechiae are blood vessels beneath the skin that produce small, red, or purple lesions on the epidermis.

7. Enlarged Liver or Spleen: The accumulation of blood cells may occasionally result in the enlargement of the liver or spleen.

Analytical Procedures For Aplastic Anemia

1. Complete Blood Count (CBC): When diagnosing aplastic anemia, a CBC is frequently the initial test administered. It determines the

platelet, red blood, and white blood cell counts in the blood.

2. Bone Marrow Biopsy: A bone marrow biopsy requires the use of a probe to remove a sample of bone marrow from the hip bone. A microscopic examination of the sample is subsequently conducted to determine the quantity and state of blood-forming cells.

3. A peripheral blood smear is an evaluation of the quantity, shape, and size of blood cells through a microscopic examination of a blood sample. Observations of irregularities in the blood smear may offer supplementary insights that aid in the diagnosis of aplastic anemia.

4. Flow cytometry is an analytical method employed to determine the attributes of specific cells, encompassing their dimensions, morphology, and surface protein composition. It has the

potential to facilitate the differentiation of various bone marrow disorders.

5. Cytogenetic testing is a procedure that examines the chromosomes of cells extracted from a sample of bone marrow to detect any mutations or genetic abnormalities that could potentially be linked to aplastic anemia.

6. Response to Immunosuppressive Therapy: Aplastic anemia may be confirmed as a diagnosis in certain instances based on the patient's response to immunosuppressive therapy, which consists of medications that inhibit the immune system to avert additional bone marrow injury.

Overall, aplastic anemia is a multifaceted hematological disorder characterized by a wide array of risk factors, symptoms, and diagnostic methodologies. Improving prognoses and averting complications is contingent upon the timely identification and suitable treatment of this condition.

The Categorization Of Aplastic Anemia

Aplastic anemia is an uncommon and critical medical condition distinguished by an insufficiency of all blood cell types, which arises from the inadequate production of these cells by the bone marrow. It is critical to comprehend its phases and classifications to administer effective management and treatment.

1. Aplastic anemia may be acquired rather than inherited, signifying that it may develop gradually as a result of exposure to contaminants, infections, or autoimmune disorders, among other things. Alternatively, the condition may be inherited through the transmission of genetic mutations from parents.

2. Clinical classification of aplastic anemia is determined by the degree of severity exhibited by the deficiency in red blood cells. Typically, this is ascertained through the analysis of platelet, hemoglobin, and white blood cell counts. Radiating from moderate to severe, severity is frequently classified as:

VSAA stands for very severe aplastic anemia.

SAA is severe aplastic anemia.

MAA stands for moderate aplastic anemia.

MIA is mild aplastic anemia.

3. Etiology-based Classification: Aplastic anemia is classified under this system according to its fundamental cause, which may include:

• Idiopathic aplastic anemia: Indisputably causing the condition.

Secondary aplastic anemia is induced by various factors, including radiation therapy, infection, exposure to pollutants, specific medications, infections (e.g., hepatitis, HIV), or autoimmune diseases.

The Progression Of Aplastic Anemia

Frequently, the degree of bone marrow suppression and the severity of symptoms are utilized to classify the phases of aplastic anemia. These phases consist of:

1. Early Stage: Patients may exhibit minimal or no symptoms during the initial phases. Although blood tests may detect a decrease in one or more blood cell types, there is no substantial impairment in the overall function of the bone marrow.

2. Intermediate Stage: As the disease advances, individuals may manifest more conspicuous symptoms as a result of additional inhibition of

bone marrow function. Anemia, heightened vulnerability to infections, and propensity for hemorrhaging may manifest.

3. Advanced Stage: Bone marrow function is profoundly impaired during the advanced phases of aplastic anemia, resulting in a substantial depletion of all blood cell types. Life-threatening complications, including severe infections, uncontrolled hemorrhage, and symptoms of severe anemia, pose a significant risk to patients.

A comprehensive comprehension of the categorization and progression of aplastic anemia is critical to ascertain suitable therapeutic approaches and forecast the prognosis of patients.

CHAPTER THREE

Alternatives To Aplastic Anemia Treatment

Aplastic anemia is treated with the following objectives: restoration of normal blood cell production, symptom relief, and enhancement of the patient's quality of life. Depending on the severity of the disease, the patient's age, general health, and additional variables, treatment options may differ. Frequent treatment modalities consist of:

1. In instances of benign illness or when patients do not meet the criteria for more aggressive therapeutic approaches, supportive care strategies may be implemented to alleviate symptoms and handle complications. This may involve platelet transfusions to control hemorrhage or blood transfusions to rectify anemia.

2. Immunosuppressive therapy may be advised for patients diagnosed with moderate to severe aplastic anemia who do not meet the criteria to undergo bone marrow transplantation. Medications such as anti-thymocyte globulin (ATG) and cyclosporine are utilized in this therapy to inhibit the immune system and halt the progression of autoimmune-mediated bone marrow cell destruction.

3. A prospective remedy for severe or very severe aplastic anemia in eligible patients with a suitable donor and allogeneic hematopoietic stem cell transplantation (HSCT) is possible. By infusing healthy stem cells from a compatible donor into the dysfunctional bone marrow, this procedure restores normal blood cell production.

4. Experimental Therapies: When standard treatments prove to be ineffective or unattainable, clinical trials may provide patients with access to experimental therapies. Potential treatments for aplastic anemia patients may consist of novel

pharmaceuticals, gene therapy techniques, or alternative transplant approaches.

Aplastic anemia treatment is determined by several variables, including the severity of the disease, the age of the patient, his or her general health, and the availability of suitable donors for transplantation. It is frequently imperative to employ a multidisciplinary approach that encompasses hematologists, transplant specialists, and supportive care teams to deliver comprehensive care for individuals living with this arduous condition.

Medications Employed In The Treatment Of Aplastic Anemia

Aplastic anemia is frequently managed with a variety of medications that suppress the immune system, promote the production of blood cells, or alleviate associated symptoms. Whether administered individually or in combination, these drugs may be modified to suit the patient's individual requirements and response to therapy. **Some medications that are frequently prescribed include:**

1. Anti-thymocyte Globulin (ATG): ATG is a human or animal-derived polyclonal antibody formulation used to reduce the destruction of bone marrow cells in aplastic anemia and suppress the immune system. Constantly administered in conjunction with other immunosuppressive agents, it constitutes a component of the prevailing treatment protocol.

2. Cyclosporine, an immunosuppressive medication, functions by impeding the functionality of specific immune cells. This mechanism of action effectively mitigates the autoimmune assault on the bone marrow associated with aplastic anemia. It is frequently administered in conjunction with ATG to induce immunosuppression.

3. Growth Factors: To induce the generation of red blood cells and white blood cells, erythropoietin and granulocyte-colony stimulating factor (G-CSF), respectively, are pharmaceutical agents that may be administered to patients diagnosed with aplastic anemia. By reducing the risk of infections and alleviating symptoms of anemia, these drugs can be of assistance.

4. Certain patients diagnosed with aplastic anemia may be prescribed androgens (e.g., danazol) to increase blood cell counts and stimulate the production of red blood cells. They are, nevertheless, generally reserved for patients who are ineligible for more aggressive therapies or who have failed to respond to alternative treatments.

5. Antibiotics and antifungal agents: Due to their low white blood cell counts, patients with aplastic anemia have an increased risk of developing infections. Therapeutically or prophylactically, antibiotics and antifungal agents may be

prescribed to treat or prevent infections and lower the likelihood of complications.

6. Transfusion Support: Red blood cell and platelet transfusions are frequently administered to patients with severe aplastic anemia to manage symptoms of anemia and hemorrhage. Long-term dependence on transfusions, on the other hand, may result in complications including iron excess and alloimmunization.

Aplastic anemia medication and treatment regimen selection is contingent on several variables, including disease severity, age of the patient, comorbidities, and previous therapeutic responses. It is critical to maintain vigilant observation and consistent communication with a hematologist or specialist in bone marrow disorders to maximize treatment efficacy and effectively handle possible adverse effects or complications.

CHAPTER FOUR

Management And Supportive Care For Aplastic Anemia

Supportive care and management are integral components of aplastic anemia treatment. Treatment aims to mitigate symptoms, avert complications, and enhance the quality of life in its entirety. Key elements of supportive care and management include the following:

1. Regular blood transfusions are frequently necessary for patients diagnosed with severe aplastic anemia to replenish compromised blood cells and mitigate symptoms including fatigue, frailty, and dyspnea. Frequent transfusions may, nevertheless, result in adverse effects including iron overload and alloimmunization.

2. Hematopoietic Stem Cell Transplantation (HSCT): By substituting healthy stem cells from a compatible donor for defective bone marrow, HSCT offers eligible patients the possibility of a cure. HSCT is generally administered to younger patients who have a suitable donor and are diagnosed with severe or very severe aplastic anemia.

3. Immunosuppressive therapy reduces the autoimmune attack on the bone marrow through the administration of medications that suppress the immune system. Cyclosporine and antithymocyte globulin (ATG) are normal immunosuppressive agents. This method is frequently applied to patients who are ineligible for HSCT or lack a suitable donor.

4. Antibiotics and Antifungal Medications: Due to their low white blood cell counts, patients with aplastic anemia are at an increased risk of contracting infections.

Antifungal and prophylactic antibiotics may therefore be prescribed to avert bacterial and fungal infections.

5. Growth Factors: In certain patients diagnosed with aplastic anemia, recombinant growth factors (G-CSF) and erythropoietin (EPO) may be administered to stimulate the production of white blood cells and red blood cells, respectively.

6. The implementation of supportive care and routine monitoring of clinical symptoms and blood counts is critical to evaluate the advancement of the disease and the effectiveness of treatment. In addition to nutritional support, pain management, and psychosocial assistance, supportive care measures are crucial for symptom management and quality of life enhancement.

Adverse Reactions And Complications Of Aplastic Anemia

Aplastic anemia is associated with a range of complications and adverse effects, the severity of which can differ based on the extent of bone marrow dysfunction and the efficacy of therapeutic interventions. The following are frequent complications and adverse effects:

1. Anemia is a condition that arises from a decrease in the production of red blood cells. It is distinguished by manifestations including fatigue, weakness, vertigo, and dyspnea. Blood transfusions may be necessary to mitigate symptoms and enhance oxygen delivery to tissues in cases of severe anemia.

2. Neutropenia, characterized by decreased levels of white blood cells, elevates the susceptibility to bacterial infections, specifically those affecting the respiratory system, gastrointestinal tract, and

epidermis. A patient with neutropenia who develops a fever is deemed to be in critical medical condition and necessitates immediate assessment and antibiotic intervention.

3. Thrombocytopenia, an etiology characterized by reduced platelet production, may contribute to an elevated susceptibility to hemorrhaging and bruising. Minor injuries may result in nosebleeds, gingival bleeding, simple bruising, or prolonged bleeding in patients. Transfusions of platelets might be required to manage or prevent episodes of hemorrhage.

4. Patients with aplastic anemia are at an increased risk of contracting infections as a result of their compromised immune function and diminished white blood cell counts. Infections caused by bacteria, viruses, and fungi are prevalent. Infections must be promptly diagnosed and treated to prevent complications and enhance prognoses.

5.   Hemorrhage: Patients   with   severe thrombocytopenia are at an increased risk of experiencing spontaneous bleeding, which can present itself in various ways, including mucosal bleeding (e.g., nosebleeds, gingival bleeding, gastrointestinal bleeding), ecchymosis (bruising), or petechiae (tiny red or purple patches on the skin). If not addressed immediately, bleeding can be fatal.

6. Quality of Life and Fatigue: A prevalent manifestation of aplastic anemia, chronic fatigue can have a substantial detrimental effect on the quality of life of affected individuals. The emotional toll of living with a chronic illness, frequent medical appointments, and anemia can all contribute to the exacerbation of fatigue. It is essential to implement supportive care measures, including sufficient rest, nutritional assistance, and psychosocial support, to combat fatigue and enhance the quality of life.

In summary, aplastic anemia is an intricate hematologic disorder distinguished by a failure of the bone marrow and an insufficiency in the production of red blood cells. The overarching goals of supportive care and management strategies are to mitigate symptoms, avert complications, and enhance the quality of life for individuals who are impacted. A multidisciplinary approach comprising hematologists, infectious disease specialists, and supportive care providers is imperative for maximizing outcomes and effectively managing the complications linked to this condition. This entails diligent observation, timely intervention, and close monitoring.

CHAPTER FIVE

Outlook And Prognosis For Patients With Aplastic Anemia

Aplastic anemia is an uncommon yet critical hematological condition distinguished by insufficient production of red blood cells, white blood cells, and platelets by the bone marrow. A reduction in the production of blood cells may result in the manifestation of symptoms including fatigue, dyspnea, heightened vulnerability to infections, and excessive bleeding or injuries. In addition to learning the prognosis and outlook for patients with aplastic anemia, it is critical to implement coping mechanisms and adopt a healthy lifestyle to effectively manage this condition.

1. Severity Variability: Aplastic anemia patients may have a wide-ranging prognosis, contingent upon several factors including the condition's

severity, age of initiation, treatment response, and the existence of concurrent health conditions.

2. Aplastic anemia may be managed via a range of therapeutic strategies, including bone marrow transplantation, immunosuppressive therapy, and blood transfusions. The prognosis is substantially impacted by the degree to which these treatments boost blood cell counts and general health.

3. Treatment Response: Certain patients exhibit favorable outcomes following initial treatments, as evidenced by notable enhancements in blood cell counts and alleviation of symptoms. Others, however, may be afflicted with a strain of the disease that is more resistant to treatment, necessitating alternative or continuous therapies.

4. Complications: Patients diagnosed with aplastic anemia face the potential for complications including infections, bleeding disorders, and secondary malignancies,

notwithstanding the efficacy of their treatment. Consequences of these complications may include a decline in prognosis and quality of life.

5. Prospects for the Future: Numerous individuals afflicted with aplastic anemia have the potential to attain sustained remission and lead gratifying existences with the aid of suitable medical interventions and care. Consistent surveillance by medical professionals is critical for the management of the condition and identification of potential complications or relapse.

6. Prognostic Factors: Age at diagnosis, severity of bone marrow failure, and response to treatment are examples of variables that can be utilized to forecast the prognosis of individuals diagnosed with aplastic anemia. A worse prognosis may be observed in patients with extensive aplastic anemia or those who do not exhibit a satisfactory response to treatment.

7. Quality of Life: Although aplastic anemia can present considerable obstacles, numerous patients' quality of life has been enhanced by developments in supportive therapies and medical care. The provision of comprehensive healthcare services, emotional support, and symptom management resources has the potential to improve the prognosis for those affected by this condition.

Coping Mechanisms And Lifestyle Choices For Aplastic Anemia

1. A balanced diet, which is abundant in vitamins, minerals, and iron, is critical for maintaining optimal health and effectively managing the symptoms associated with aplastic anemia. Patients should incorporate a sizable portion of whole cereals, fruits, vegetables, and lean proteins into their diet.

2. Consistent Physical Activity: Participating in consistent physical activity can contribute to

enhanced energy levels, improved circulation, and fortified immune function. However, before beginning an exercise regimen, individuals with aplastic anemia should consult their healthcare provider due to the potential dangers associated with specific activities.

3. The management of stress is crucial for preserving mental and emotional health in the face of chronic illness. Yoga, deep breathing exercises, and mindfulness meditation are all examples of stress-reduction practices that can be utilized to alleviate anxiety and encourage relaxation.

4. Aplastic anemia patients are at an increased risk of contracting infections as a result of their compromised immune systems. Maintaining current vaccinations, practicing good hygiene, and avoiding contact with individuals who are ailing can all contribute to a decreased risk of contracting an illness.

5. Medication Management It is critical to effectively manage aplastic anemia so that patients adhere to their prescribed medications and treatment plans. Patients must collaborate closely with their healthcare team to gain a comprehensive understanding of their treatment regimen and any possible adverse effects.

6. Pacing Activities: Patients with aplastic anemia must prioritize rest and energy conservation due to the prevalence of fatigue as a symptom of the condition. One can prevent overexertion by breaking down tasks into manageable segments, delegating responsibilities whenever feasible, and scheduling regular rest periods throughout the day.

7. Social Support: Establishing a robust support system comprising healthcare professionals, family members, and acquaintances can offer invaluable practical aid and emotional solace in managing the difficulties associated with aplastic anemia. Patients may also find solace in online

communities or support groups comprised of individuals who share their struggles.

8. Consistent Medical Monitoring: It is critical to schedule routine follow-up consultations with healthcare providers to assess the efficacy of treatments, monitor blood cell counts, and address any emerging symptoms or concerns. Maintaining transparent lines of communication with healthcare providers is crucial for ensuring that patients diagnosed with aplastic anemia receive the necessary care and support throughout their condition.

Through comprehension of the prognosis, adoption of health-conscious lifestyle behaviors, and implementation of efficacious coping mechanisms, those afflicted with aplastic anemia can maximize their standard of living and effectively navigate the obstacles that accompany this uncommon blood disorder.

Summary

In summary, Aplastic Anemia is an uncommon yet critical medical condition distinguished by insufficient erythrocyte production in the bone marrow. It is hypothesized that exposure to specific substances, radiation, medications, and viral infections all play a role in its development, although the precise causes remain unknown. Manifestations of the condition may include increased vulnerability to infections, uncontrolled hemorrhage, fatigue, and frailty.

Obtaining an early diagnosis via bone marrow biopsies and blood testing is critical for effective management. Depending on the severity of the condition, potential treatments include bone marrow transplants, blood transfusions, and medications that stimulate the production of blood cells. In addition, preventative measures against infections and supportive care, including antibiotics, are critical.

Prognosis exhibits significant variability among individuals, as certain may benefit from treatment and attain remission, whereas others may confront chronic or relapsing conditions that necessitate continuous medical supervision. It is impossible to overstate the psychological and emotional toll on patients and their families; therefore, comprehensive support systems and counseling services are required.

Advancements in medical research present the potential for enhanced comprehension and control of Aplastic Anemia, underscoring the criticality of ongoing financial support for scientific pursuits that seek to improve the well-being of individuals impacted by this disorder.

By integrating healthcare providers, researchers, and support networks into a multidisciplinary framework, significant progress can be achieved in improving the prognosis and standard of living for those afflicted with Aplastic Anemia.

THE END

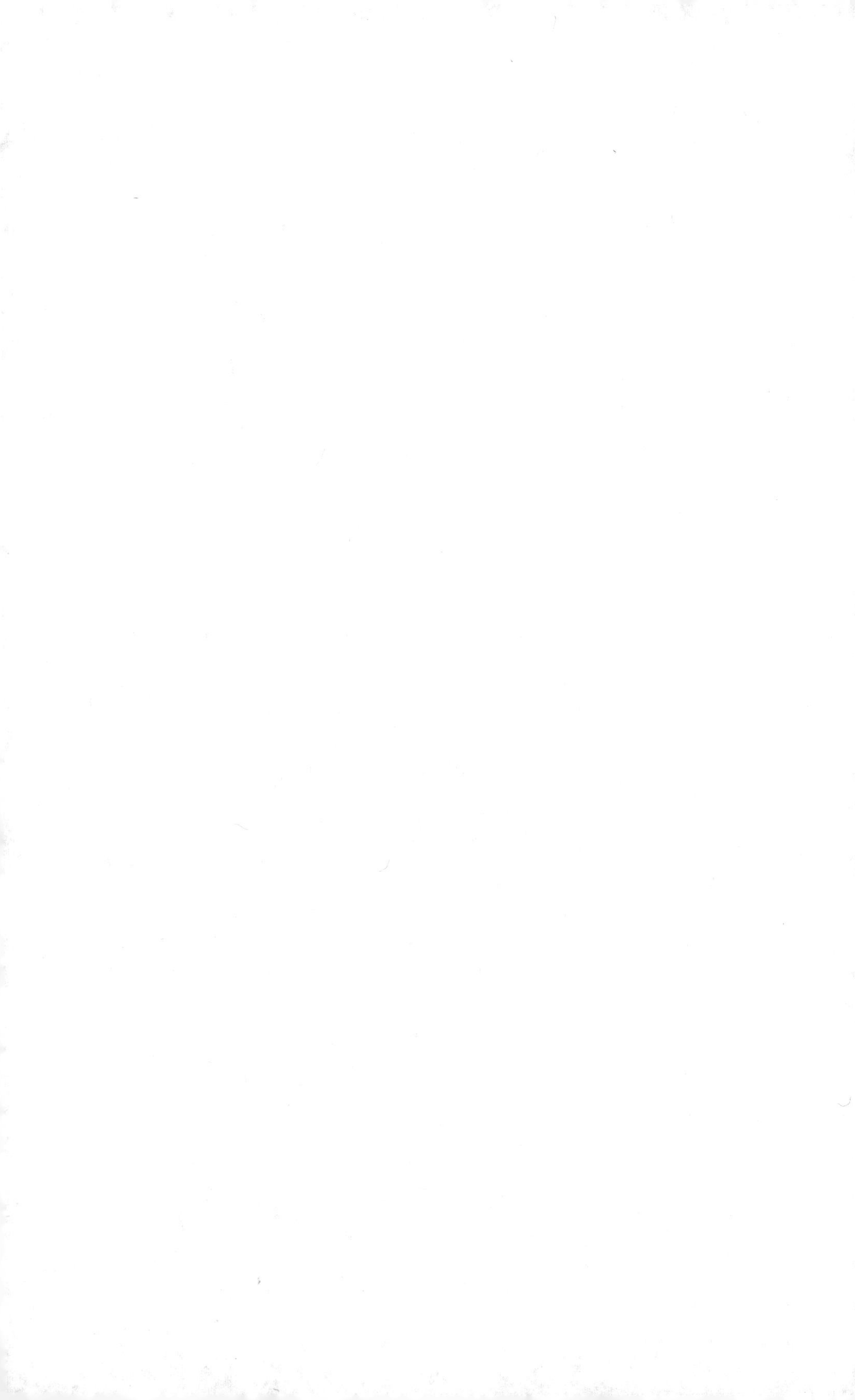

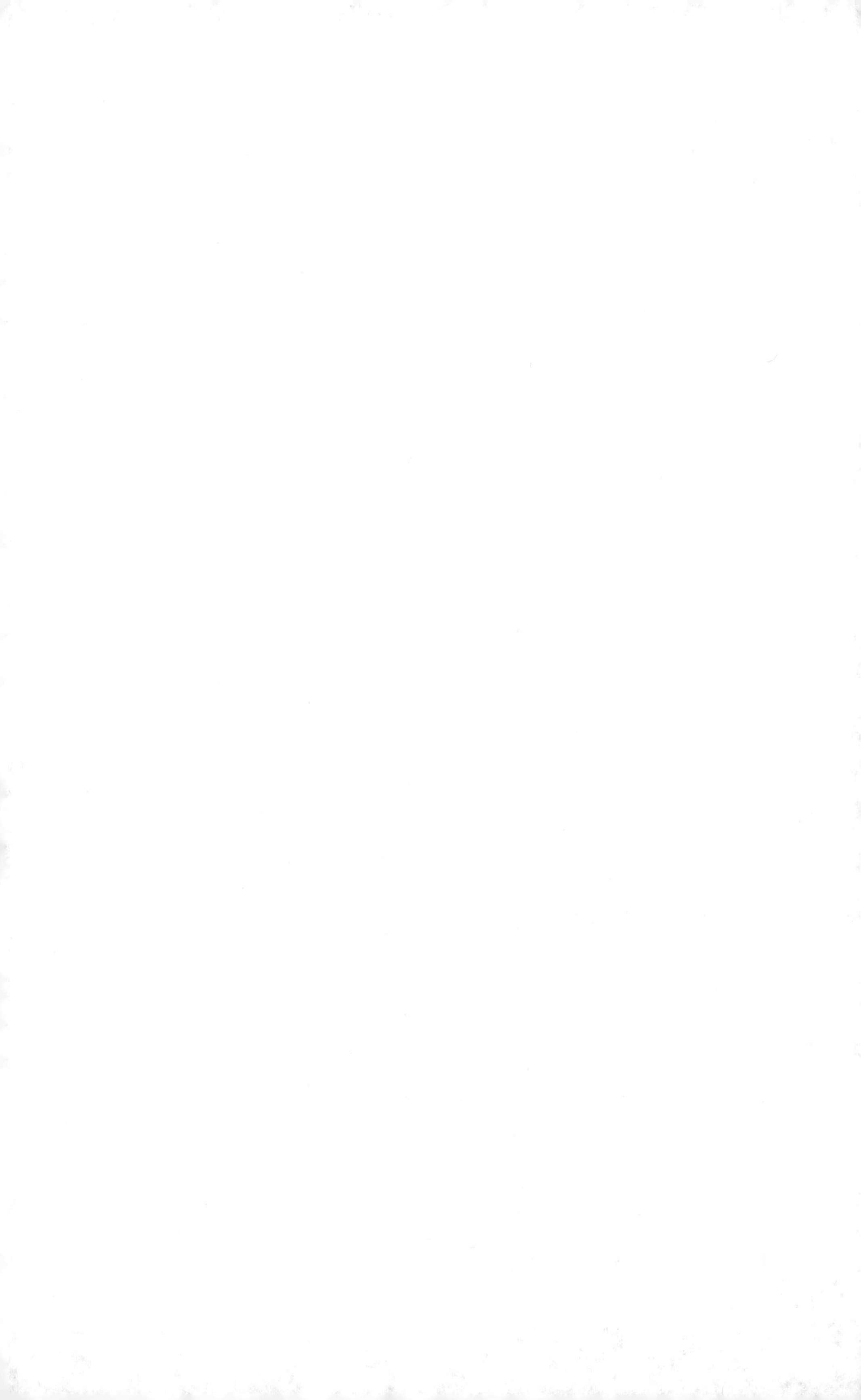

www.ingramcontent.com/pod-product-compliance
Lightning Source LLC
Chambersburg PA
CBHW061312250726
48653CB00002B/902